Relieving Stress Through Gardening

The Natural Way to Mental Relaxation
And
Healthy Produce

RON KNESS

Contents

Introduction

For years, men and women have seen an alarming increase in the amount of stress they incur over a typical work week. With both parents working, and many struggling to afford and maintain a typical household, anxiety soars.

Even children are experiencing more stress now than in the past, unable to cope with the normal routines of childhood, mixed with a strong tie to technology and never-ending stimulation.

It's no wonder that prescription medications are on the rise, and more people are seeking counseling or other therapies to help them achieve a sense of peace and calm. But amid all of this bad news, there's positive news on the horizon, also!

Whenever gardening is mentioned, it can be overwhelming for some individuals. They picture a large plot of land filled with rows and rows of vegetables. The task can sound more daunting than stress relieving.

But once you learn how many different variations of gardening there are, and how many health benefits it provides you, you'll be on the fast track to becoming a gardening enthusiast, and it will all be done without any hesitation or fear of being able to handle what all it entails.

Gardening is going to help you from head to toe, inside out – and it won't just be a benefit to you personally, but to your loved ones as well. Your bounty can help provide benefits for your spouse, your children, and anyone you share the harvest with.

First, you have to understand exactly what all can happen when you start growing your own plants. That can be fruits, vegetables, herbs or even flowers. It's going to assist you in getting a good night's sleep, in building a stronger immune system, and in helping you handle stress better.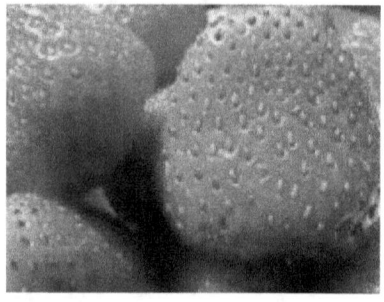

You'll want to start relying on this natural method of getting rid of stress instead of popping pills if the matter isn't warranted. Of course, your doctor will be beneficial in helping you make this decision, but it's worth testing the gardening process to see how much it impacts your stress levels.

And if your weight or nutrition habits contribute to your anxiety, then gardening can pinpoint those problems and help eliminate them, too. Fresh, beautiful vegetables and fruits can improve your health and help you whittle your waist as you engage in the process. Let's start by taking a look at the problem with stress relievers that come from a factory, and not nature.

The Problem with Unnatural Stress Relievers

If you have stress in your life, you're not alone. There are millions who suffer from stress. Unfortunately, the go-to answer seems to be to rely on medication in an effort to relieve the stress. The problem with using this approach to deal with stress is that the medication is a temporary fix.

Stress Relief Isn't All You Get with Medicine

It's true there are numerous medications on the market today designed to treat stress. You can get a prescription from your doctor today and, depending on the medication prescribed, you can feel relief from the stress almost instantly.

That's what most people focus on. The quick relief only and not what else they might be introducing into their body. When you get a prescription, you always get a pharmacy information insert with it.

Most people don't even bother to read those. But this information is there for a reason. It's there to warn consumers about the side effects of taking certain pills. You'll always see the disclaimer that the doctor has decided that the benefits of the medicine far outweigh any side effects.

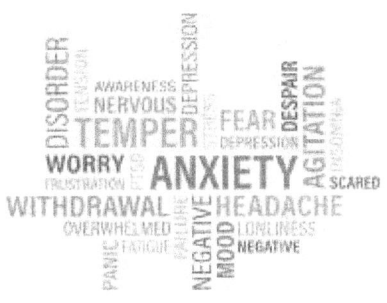

Which doesn't sound so bad, so most people go ahead and take it. Then comes actually having to live with the side effects and those can be a deal breaker. These well-known medications are known as anti-anxiety drugs.

They're designed to work on your nervous system. They're powerful drugs that can work quickly to make you feel calm. But the problem is that because they impact your nervous system, you won't function at 100%.

The medications can cause you to feel sleepy during the day and can also rob you of energy. You'll feel lethargic as if you're a beat behind. Other side effects of the medications include slowing down your ability to react.

While that might not seem like a big deal, it can impact your ability to drive a car as well as react in any emergency situation. Because the medications affect the brain, you may start to notice that you have trouble speaking clearly.

You won't be able to concentrate as well and you can experience a lack of clarity in your thinking. Some people refer to this as "brain fog." Taking medicine for stress relief can give you problems walking because it can cause you to feel like the room is spinning.

You might experience problems with dizziness and feel like you're going to pass out. Other side effects include things like trouble recalling events due to struggling with memory retention.

You might also feel sick to your stomach and have a loss of appetite. Some people also experience problems with comprehension and struggling with feelings of depression is also common on stress relief medications.

Dependency Can Be a Problem

Like many other types of drugs, anti-anxiety medications do have the potential to become addictive. In fact, one of the known side effects of many stress relieving drugs is developing a dependency on the medicine in order to function.

This happens because the medications give you those feel good sensations or reward pathways within the brain that you would get from taking drugs like heroin. You might not have a substance abuse history in your family and you might be someone who has never become dependent on a drug in your life.

However, because of the way anti-anxiety medication works on the brain, you can easily cross the line because over time, the effectiveness of the medication lowers. So what happens then is that people end up taking more and more of the drug because their tolerance level has increased.

They have to take a higher dosage of the medication in order to get any relief. This is why most anti-anxiety prescriptions are written for short term use only and are heavily monitored by doctors.

Over time, what happens is that anti-anxiety drugs have been known to build up in your system. When that occurs, you actually end up with too much of the drug in your body. This can lead to a state of being medicated beyond your body's ability to metabolize it fast enough.

What's worse is that when your doctor has to raise your dosage, the likelihood of having a buildup in your body increases as well. People who are on even small dosages of anti-anxiety medications used to treat stress can end up with numerous side effects.

These side effects can give off the same symptoms you would see in someone who had too much alcohol to drink. You would find it difficult to function in your professional and private life.

Signs of dependency on anti-anxiety medications are pretty easy to spot. You'll feel tired and won't have the energy to do much. Feeling confused and unable to concentrate are signs of dependence.

So is developing trouble walking without shuffling or stumbling when you move. Red or glassy eyes that appear vacant is a sign. So is trouble speaking and having trouble understanding simple questions.

Changes in mood or sudden mood swings are yet more signs of dependency. You become easily irritated and feel upset at the thought of not being able to take the medication.

Being unable to sleep, or feeling wired or edgy, is also a sign of dependency. Going from doctor to another in an effort to get more of the pills is also a sign you've become addicted.

On top of becoming physically dependent on stress relieving medications, you can also become psychologically dependent on them. When this happens, it's easier to rely on the medicine rather than try to make changes to eliminate stress.

Medicating for Stress Relief Numbs You

You can't take medication without experiencing changes in the way that you think and feel. Anti-anxiety medications for treating stress are known to cause changes in how you feel and cope with life.

If you're someone who has struggled with stress, you might feel that being numb would be better than feeling everything you're feeling. However, the medication can make it difficult for you to deal with more than whatever caused your stress.

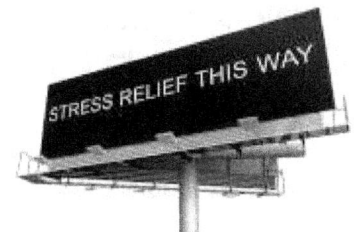

When you take pills in the anti-anxiety class of medications, they don't simply make you stop caring about whatever was stressing you out. They make you stop caring about a lot of things.

You'll find it difficult to connect personally. You won't care what goes on in your family, not because your feelings toward friends and loved ones has changed, but because the medication has changed the way your brain receives and responds to emotional information.

Taking medication isn't effective for stress relief because it binds your emotions. You won't feel sad. You won't feel happy or excited. Nothing will give you pain but you won't have pleasurable feelings, either.

In fact, you won't feel at all. You simply go through the motions of living life that you're not really experiencing. The medicine prevents you from finding effective stress relief and keeps you from reaching a resolution because it acts as a smothering cover.

You don't feel the emotions that you once felt with stress so you think you're okay now. But the problem is that you can't move forward when you've been numbed to the stress. You're still stuck in the same situation, in the same place with the same stress, but you don't feel it so you don't deal with it.

What's going on is that the medication acts as a "bridge out" mechanism preventing you from crossing over the stress to get to the other side of it. This is the point where many people develop the habit of pretending they feel happy or other emotions and they often don't even realize they're doing that.

When it's time to get off the drugs, you'll end up feeling worse when you do finally stop the medication than you did when you first started taking it because the reaction and symptoms you had to the stress will still be there.

It's always best to find a natural way to deal with whatever stress is going on in your life rather than relying on any type of chemical solution. You want something that will help you to relax and relieve stress that you can turn to over and over again that won't end up numbing you.

Medicating Addresses Symptoms Not Root Causes

Everyone experiences stress at some point in his or her life. Stress can be big or small and can impact your life to the point it can become a struggle just to get through a day. There is a big misunderstanding about exactly what stress is.

When people are dealing with it, they believe that it's a condition like a disease that can easily be treated if they just take some medicine. But stress is not a condition. It's not a disease.

That's why medication isn't the answer. Stress is a collection of symptoms. It's the symptoms that medicine targets. Stress can manifest itself in a variety of ways and no two people will feel it the same way.

You might feel anxious or worried. You might have fears and not really understand them. You might experience upset stomach and nausea. You might struggle with insomnia or go to the opposite end and sleep way too much.

All of those are merely signs that the stress in your life is showing up physically. It can show up emotionally, too. You can find yourself becoming increasingly short tempered. Little things might irritate you or cause you to blow up at others.

You can have bouts of crying and not know exactly why you're crying. When some people realize that what they're going through is because of stress, they end up seeking a medication solution.

Unfortunately, it's not really a solution. Treating stress with medication is a pause. If you want to cure stress or reduce it in your life, you must address the root cause that's behind the stress.

Sometimes this can be related to your job or to relationship struggles. To figure it out, you just need to stop and reflect. Ask yourself why you feel like your stomach is in knots or why you dread facing a situation or someone.

Of course, identifying the root cause is the first step to take toward eliminating it. Once you know what's behind the stress, you can get it out of your life or learn how to manage it properly.

But in the meantime, you'll need an outlet to find relief from the stress. Otherwise, the symptoms will feel too overwhelming to deal with. You have to give yourself a break both physically and emotionally from stress.

What many doctors suggest for that for people who want to avoid taking anti-anxiety medications is to get involved in some type of hobby that's calming.

Everyone will have a different idea of what interests them.

Medicating Is Expensive, Inconvenient, and Stressful

Regardless of what type of way you pay for your medications, it can be expensive to buy medications for dealing with stress. Even buying generic medications can be costly. With some types of health insurance, you can usually get medicine to treat stress at a pretty decent price.

However, not all insurance plans will cover medications for stress that aren't specifically labeled as for an anxiety condition. Since stress is not an anxiety disorder, your doctor won't treat it as such.

If you have insurance, regardless of which medication your doctor might decide is best for you, your insurance company has a list of preferred ones. You could be forced to take a generic or a completely different type than what your doctor first chose.

If you try one medication and have a reaction to it, you'll have to stop taking it. Then, it can become inconvenient to have to go back and get a different script. Some medications used to treat stress aren't able to be called in.

Depending on what they are, federal laws prohibit some from being routed electronically from your doctor's office to the pharmacy due to their addictive nature. Plus, your doctor's office might have a policy about calling in a new medicine if the first one didn't work.

You'll have to go into the office and pick up another script. If you have medication limitations per month on your insurance, this can count against you if it's not properly booted out of the system.

Taking medication to treat stress can actually turn around and cause stress. You can't take certain ones with alcohol because they can be fatal when taken that way. You can't take some of them with other medications.

It can also be stressful if you end up losing, spilling, or accidentally running out of the script. You can't simply quit stress relieving drugs cold turkey. You have to slowly wean off of them using the tapering method.

Depending on how long you've been on them, it can take months to taper off. Even then you still run the risk of having to deal with withdrawal symptoms once you stop taking them.

It's better to find more natural methods to relieve the symptoms of stress rather than to rely to medications that can cause side effects and prevent you from dealing with stress in a healthier way.

How Gardening Helps You Get a Good Night's Sleep

Among the many benefits of gardening, the boost in your ability to get a good night's sleep is one of the best. Sleep has a paramount impact on your quality of life – if you don't get enough sleep you may not be as alert and focused the next day.

Other perks of gardening include keeping your body flexible, the bounty you enjoy (whether flowers or food) and creating a beautiful spot to boost your sense of well-being.

There's also something to be said for getting in touch with the earth. We generally live "dirt-free" lives – almost sterile in nature. But playing in the earth can be a good thing when it relaxes you and gets you ready for a restorative night's sleep.

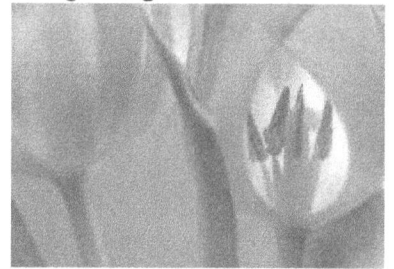

Even if you're limited to gardening in pots, the act can have a huge impact in keeping your stress levels low and improving your mental and physical states. It's a leisure activity that most can join in and create a beautiful and happy place.

The Scientific Explanation

The scientific explanation of how gardening can help you get a good night's sleep is multi-faceted and addresses all the senses – touch, taste, smell, sight and sound.

The mental and physical health boost that gardening brings into your life is well documented as a positive influence to cultivate in your lifestyle.

If you're subject to bouts of mood swings and/or depression, gardening is proven to provide major improvement by addressing all the senses in a positive way. For example, digging in the dirt, tasting the bounty that you helped to grow, smelling fresh earth or plants, viewing the beauty of a well-tended garden and listening to the wind, chirp of birds and other garden sounds can help you relax and lift your mood.

Gardening is an activity that relaxes all of the senses in such a unique manner that you can't find elsewhere. Studies indicate that people who are diagnosed with depression, mood swings and bipolar disorder and spent up to six hours per week gardening flowers or vegetables show intense improvement in their symptoms.

These people reported much improved lifestyle and better habits and much more luck in getting a good night's sleep. Plus, scientists have found that a harmless bacteria (Mycobacterium) found in soil has the power to help release serotonin in parts of the brain having to do with mood and cognitive functioning.

While not as powerful as the medications sometimes prescribed for depression and insomnia, gardening does put back some help to your immune system that's quite lacking in our environment of today.

The exercise you get from gardening is also a scientific factor in helping you finally achieve a good night's sleep. The fresh air and sunshine are like a powerful tonic on your immune system and gets your blood flowing.

Gardening is an especially good exercise to choose if you're limited in movement. While it doesn't usually give you a cardiovascular workout, it does move your muscles with the digging, weeding, planting and other gardening tasks.

Stretching and most gardening tasks are low impact but are found to greatly help those who are in their senior years, have certain disabilities or those suffering from chronic pain.

Another plus to gardening exercise is that you'll more than likely stick to the program and get regular exercise because a garden takes tending and if you want to realize the most beauty and bounty from it, you'll want to keep up with the tasks.

Your brain health can be boosted with the exercise and other experiences you gain from gardening. Many seniors, faced with mental decline have found that simply walking through a garden is therapeutic.

Now, residential homes for those with memory problems are including gardens in their landscaping so the residents can enjoy a walk without fear from getting lost. That positive influence also extends to bedtime hours.

Your diet can also be a factor in how you sleep at night. Gardening makes you much more aware of your eating habits and gives you the opportunity to grow some foods you can eat.

Scientific surveys show that those who grow and eat much of their food from a garden are much more likely to eat healthier than non-gardeners. It's also a big factor in helping kids eat healthier. They're more likely to eat veggies and fruit they have a hand in growing.

The Spiritual Connection of Sleep and Gardening

To get a peaceful night's sleep, you should have spiritual peace-of-mind. You don't have to be religious to find peace – but you do have to immerse your senses in whatever makes your spirits and your mood soar.

The sense of healing and well-being that you get from being in the great outdoors can make all the difference in relaxing your body and mind so a good night's sleep is easy to come by.

Being in tune with the universe comes from your thoughts – and it's difficult to be in a bad mood when gardening – whether you're potting an array of flowers on your patio or arranging savory herbs on a window sill, your body naturally relaxes.

If you've been chained to a computer or iPhone all day or week, you'll get a new perspective on life. Gardening can clear away the trivia from your mind and provide peace from the noisy and fast-moving world we live in today.

Gardening helps to get you in tune with your search for renewal, being one with the earth and expanding our relationship with others. The seasons of gardening keep you in tune with life's cycle – being born, planting seeds, harvesting, fighting diseases and finally, dying.

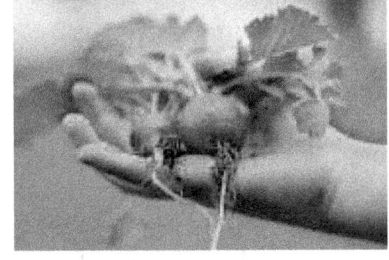

Since each and every place on earth has its own climate and geology types, you can learn about gardening experiences in various places. Gardening in Australia is very different than gardening in the United States. The hemispheres are switched and even the seasons are vastly different.

With gardening, you learn about the evolution of gardens in other parts of the world if you want and to compare it with what you're capable of in your own climate. It's a learning experience that's good for the mind and helps you become enthused about what you're doing.

When you're most happy and content is when you can get a good night's sleep without even thinking about it. Gardening is for meditation, learning, creating, touching, tasting and reveling in the wonders of nature.

How Gardening Helps Your Health – and Your Sleep Patterns

A healthy body is more apt to relax and enjoy a good night's sleep than one filled with stress, overweight, stiff and sore or on powerful medications. When your body is healthy, it's much more likely your sleep will all into healthy patterns.

Gardening burns calories – how many depends on how much work can be found in your garden. If you're tending a window herb garden, you won't likely burn as many calories as if you have a large vegetable garden outdoors.

But, there are many other gardening factors that contribute to your good health besides burning calories. For example, it may reduce the chances of developing osteoporosis in your later years.

Digging, planting and weeding or any repetitive activity requiring stretching or lifting keeps muscles and bones strong and keeps them from deteriorating so rapidly.

Gardening may also reduce the pain and inflammation of arthritis and other diseases, so a good night's sleep is easier to come by.

Known as one of nature's best stress busters, gardening is a leisure activity that should help you release stress and relax without the hassle of going to a gym to get the same results.

Those who garden were found to have lower levels of cortisol – a hormone produced by your body during stressful times. The smell of flowers and being around their beauty may also have an impact on your happiness and even improve your desire for socialization.

Children who are allowed to play in dirt during their early years are proven to have healthier immune systems that those whose parents were overly-concerned about getting dirty.

The "dirty" kids were found to have fewer instances of eczema, allergies and asthma as the years passed. Without the bother of these symptoms to wake you up constantly, you'll get a good night's sleep.

Vitamin D is one of the best reasons for gardening. Vitamin D comes most abundantly from the sun and when you're gardening, you'll love the feeling of the warm rays that add so much to your health. Just make sure you pre-plan for times you might be subjected to sunburn.

Your health is vitally important to your sleep habits. The healing and calming powers of gardening help to keep you healthy - as does the warmth of the sun on a beautiful morning.

Gardening Therapy Can Turn Your Life Around

Whether you're an outdoor or indoor gardener, the process of digging, planting and harvesting can turn your life around for the better by helping you get healthy and have a better outlook on life – and that includes getting a good night's sleep.

Your life can't be very much fun if you're sleepy and worn out when you could be having fun. Gardening indoors or outdoors is super therapy for almost all that ails you. Indoor gardens and plants bring color and much-needed oxygen into your home.

Outdoor gardening provides Vitamin D, helps you absorb calcium to your bones and keeps your body limber. Interacting with nature can also influence your mindset and your spiritual needs.

Gardening effects are restorative and help you move away from the pressures, stress and demands you may experience during the day. Try relaxing with a book or some soft music or friends in an outdoor garden you created yourself – surrounded by plants, earth, rocks, water features and color.

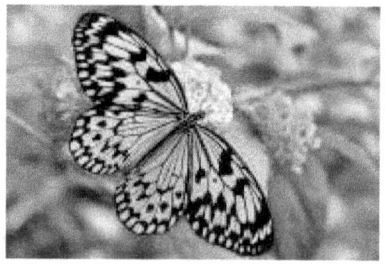

It's just a sampling of the way gardening and the results of gardening can help you get a good night's sleep. Even the plants involved with gardening can help you relax and put you in the mood for some shut eye.

Lavender, basil and mint have lovely scents for your home and garden and may even be used in your favorite recipes.

Studies also show that gardening is especially good for those who are planning surgical procedures.

The speed of recovery partially depends on your environment. If you can get out to some fresh sunshine and the sound, scent and touch of beautiful plants in your garden, you'll feel more like getting the rest you need for a full recovery.

Gardening has been compared by some therapist as a "working vacation." The rest it allows for the body and mind is like a gift of time to be by yourself and with yourself. If you're having trouble sleeping, the problem could be that your mind has no time to rest.

Stress may be interfering with every aspect of your life – and when stress is that prevalent, loss of sleep will likely occur. Gardening is a combination of exercise and manna for the mind and body.

Studies indicate that only thirty minutes per day in the garden can encourage a full eight hours of quality sleep per night. If you're having trouble sleeping, both your body and mind is trying to tell you something.

Take the hint and change your lifestyle to one that's more conducive to getting a good night's sleep. Changes such as getting more time outdoors and being more relaxed at bedtime are the best sleep aids – much better than taking prescription medications that can be harmful to your health.

Gardening can also be tonic for the soul. If you're feeling down and out, angry or frustrated when you go to bed, try a bit of gardening activity for a few minutes before retiring to see what difference it can make in the way you view your surroundings and the world.

You can open a new world by taking up gardening. Whether you have a windowsill or a large plot for your green thumb, plan carefully to plant what makes you happy, restores your senses and well-being – and helps you experience the sweet dreams you deserve.

Gardening Plays a Role in Your Stress Eating Habits

When you're under stress, it can drive you toward a lot of different behaviors. One of the behaviors that it can create is the desire to eat in ways that aren't as healthy as they should be.

And stress eating can become a habit. When you feel stressed, you want to eat and then when you eat, you feel guilty and more stressed when you eat things that aren't good for your body.

How Stress Triggers Eating

You may be familiar with how emotional stress can make you feel. It can cause anxiety, mood swings, insomnia and long term, it can lead to depression. When you're stressed, there are chemical changes that take place inside your body.

Stress causes your body to release hormones that make you crave the comfort of your favorite foods. These foods are often loaded with little in the way of nutrition but are packed with calories.

When people are under stress, it tends to make them eat more in the way of serving sizes than they would normally eat. When your life isn't under stress, your body works better to help through the use of hormones to control your appetite.

These hormones work together to make sure your desire to eat is at a healthy level. You won't have the craving to overeat. You'll experience times when you don't even feel hungry.

But that all changes when stress enters the picture and it's not your fault. There's a scientific reason that stress triggers your desire to eat. When you're under stress, whether it's short term or chronic, the body works to produce cortisol.

Just like other hormones work to keep your appetite at a healthy level, cortisol does the opposite. It prods the brain in reaction to stress to give you a signal that you need to eat in order to get some energy.

This is an automatic reaction within the body. As a result of the cortisol, it makes you hungry. It can make you crave food as the cortisol levels rise. You'll end up overeating because of this elevated hormone.

When you're not under stress, you won't have as much of the hormone present in your body. But if the stress is chronic, the cortisol levels remain at the point where you feel the need to eat more than you should and more often than you should.

What most people do when the stress hits is they reach for the foods that are packed with sugar and high in calories. This is partly due to convenience sake. These foods are usually already stocked in the pantry and we're more apt to eat whatever is on hand when we have a desire to feed the stress.

The problem is that once you eat foods that are high in fat and sugar, you experience a boomerang result. The more foods that are packed with sugar and fat that you feed your body, the more that it wants.

You can become addicted to these foods as a way of relieving stress. Even though that relief is short lived, because you feel better after eating it, the temptation to do the same thing again will be stronger.

Foods that are high in sugar can create a feel good sensation in the brain. It's because of this fact that it will be easier to eat the same unhealthy foods whenever stress increases.

The problem though with using food to try and get relief from the stress is that it always backfires. You might feel better every time you give in to stress eating, but the consequences are always there.

When you stress eat with foods that aren't healthy, you create a reward pathway that wires your brain to make eating the foods the first resort instead of trying to work toward a better solution.

The only way that you'll find relief from this behavior is to replace the foods that aren't as healthy with ones that are. Stress eaters will always go for the foods that are convenient. If you have healthier options on hand, then you can break the habit of stress eating foods that aren't good for you.

What Stress Eating Does to Your Body

If you look up funny sayings about stress, you'll find a lot of material. You'll find shirts, pillows, and décor that joke about stress. While those might be intended as humorous, it's not funny at all what stress eating can do to your body.

When you eat due to stress, you usually end up eating far more calories than your body is able to use for what it needs to run efficiently. As a result of this, weight gain usually happens.

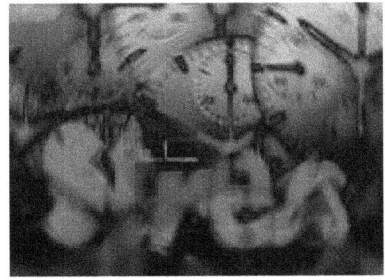

If the overeating continues for too long, you can end up gaining enough weight to push your BMI into an unhealthy level. Obesity is a well-known side effect of overeating due to stress.

When you carry this extra weight, your muscles have to work harder and you'll start to notice that your joints feel this extra weight. You can cause damage to your joints from overeating.

Stress eating can take a toll on you emotionally. Even though it might calm the stress temporarily, you'll feel guilty about it and can experience negative self-talk. Many people start to have struggles with their self-esteem due to stress eating.

When you stress eat, you learn to use the food at an emotional crutch and the desire to eat until you feel better even if you're full is often present. Stress eating can lead to problems with your vitamin and mineral levels.

Because there's a tendency to fill up on foods that are convenient but have little nutritional value rather than healthy ones, your body can become deficit in the important vitamins and minerals it needs to function well.

Consuming a diet that's high in fat and sugar can cause you to develop health problems. You can struggle with high blood pressure and run a greater risk for having a heart attack or stroke.

You can increase the risk of becoming insulin resistant which in turn damage your internal organs, causing things like a fatty liver. You also raise your risk of becoming a diabetic when you stress eat.

Your cholesterol level will also go up which can lead to potential heart disease. While there's no doubt that it's your body's own hormone release that pushes you to want to eat when you're stressed, you can't change that.

But what you can change in response to stress is what you eat. You don't have to eat the foods that will lead to weight gain and health problems. Instead, you can use stress eating to actually eat healthier if you have a way to replace the foods that aren't good for you.

Gardening Gives You Better Stress Eating Habits

The way to find a solution to unhealthy stress eating is to give yourself a better option with your food selection. Most people actually do want to eat healthy. But when it's the end of the day and you know the streets are packed with traffic and the stores are a madhouse, you'll be more resistant to want to leave your home or work to go in search of healthy eating options.

Instead, what you can do is make it easy to have good stress eating habits. That might sound strange at first, that you can indulge stress eating. It's not the eating that's the problem, it's what you eat and if you change what you eat, then stress eating isn't bad for you.

Even if you use it as a way to feel better. What you can do is to get involved with gardening. If you're thinking that gardening would raise your stress level, you'd be wrong.

Gardening is known as a relaxing hobby that offers a ton of benefits in return for the effort you do put into it. It's not like it used to be in the old days when gardening was a back breaking, all day, week in, week out affair.

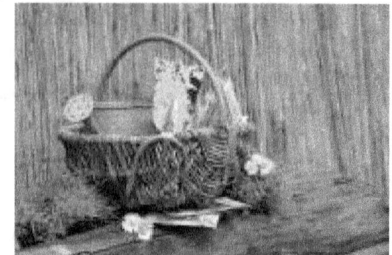

Now, there are tons of different choices you can make with gardening. You don't have to let it be something that soaks up all of your time and energy. Gardening is something that can be done easily and you'll discover that it's something you enjoy.

You can find books that will teach you about gardening from the set up all the way to the time to harvest whatever it is that you've planted. These step by step instructions can walk a beginner through it.

You can use methods like slow gardening if you want to. You can choose to plot out an area of your backyard for gardening and there are books that will teach you about the soil as well as the type of irrigation that you'll need to have in order to grow things well.

But not everyone wants to use the backyard method for gardening. If that's the case, you have options like tier planters that you can use. These planters can be placed right on a deck or on a patio and you can garden with ease.

The reason that you want to get into gardening to help you with stress eating is because you can replace the unhealthy food choices you've been making. Studies have shown that people will eat healthier if the food is readily available.

When it's something that you grow yourself, you have direct access to the healthier, home grown foods at any time. That means that you eat better than you normally would when stress eating.

Natural foods are packed with vitamins and minerals and the nutrients that you need for good health. They're much lower in both calories and fat content. So you'll be able to consume more and not gain weight like you would on a high sugar, high fat stress eating habit.

If you find that you crave sugar with stress eating, you can plant fruits that will appease your sweet tooth. Strawberries, blueberries, and melons are rich in antioxidants and vitamins and will satisfy your desire for something sweet.

You'll be able to eat without guilt and without gaining weight and causing yourself health problems. Studies have shown that one thing that people crave when they do stress eat is foods that have a crunch to them.

That's why people will eat far too many chips or crackers when they're stressed. It's not so much the food as the crunch that's associated with eating it. You can plant foods that give you the same crunch.

Foods like carrots can help you feel full while giving you the crunch you're looking for. Best of all with gardening for stress eating, is that you'll have healthier foods on hand for any chaotic moment in life.

You won't have to run out to the store when you feel the need to stress eat. You can turn to your own garden. Not only will you discover that you're eating healthier, but you'll experience the emotional and mental satisfaction that comes along with eating something that you've grown.

And another good side to gardening is that you'll be saving money on your vegetables and fruits over what you were paying at the grocery store for the unhealthy food choices.

Gardening to Help a Stress Eating Habit Can Help Your Weight

Gardening can boost the feel good hormones in your brain, which help fight against feelings associated with stress. Studies have shown that people who have a garden eat better and have fewer long term negative health effects.

Plus, another upside to gardening for stress eating is that you'll discover that instead of putting weight on, you're actually losing it instead. Most people are surprised to find that they lose inches around their waist and drop numbers on the scale through gardening.

It doesn't seem like exercise because it's a fun, fairly easy hobby to get into. The best part is that gardening isn't something that requires you drag yourself to an exercise club, wear workout gear or pay for a membership.

It's all convenient and very low cost. You just have to buy the seeds or the starter plants. You can get started with gardening through container gardening, window box gardening, indoor or outdoor gardening.

There are so many different types of foods you can plant, too. When you're involved in growing a gardening, you get exercise in a variety of ways. It's good for any body type and any weight because the exercising is all low key and low 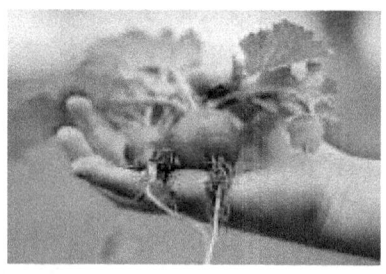 impact so you won't feel it in your joints.

Picking up the plants to move them from a pot to the soil works the upper body. As you work on transplanting, you're working out core muscles as well.

Lifting bags of soil to add to the garden plot is part of a garden workout.

So is raking the soil and digging in it to plant items. There's also weeding, which is a repetitive exercise that relaxes both the mind and the body. You can burn calories in your garden by mulching and other tasks required to keep a garden productive.

Some foods require more effort to grow than other foods and that also contributes to weight loss. If you're doing more physical aspects of gardening such as hoeing, this is considered a moderate workout and you can end up burning as much as 300 calories for every hour that you're hoeing.

You'll end up giving your muscles strength from all the activity as well as toning them. Gardening calms the mind, too – which, in turn reduces stress and lowers cortisol. When the cortisol is lowered, you'll also have less of a drive to turn to food for comfort.

Use Gardening to Achieve Mental Relaxation

Gardening is known for many things. Besides growing your own foods and being able to eat healthier, the hobby can help you achieve mental relaxation. Many studies have shown that people who spend time outdoors engaged in gardening have a lower stress and anxiety level than people who don't.

One of the thoughts behind this is that gardening provides a form of exercise which helps with mental focus and relaxes the body. The act of gardening is known for tranquility because you're spending time in nature.

The Benefits of Being in Nature

Ever notice that when you're inside all day, you experience a feeling of being cooped up? And if you're inside too much, you feel restless and you may experience some downswings in how you feel emotionally.

It happens because you can't find the same kind of peace inside that you can find when you spend time with nature. When you're outside, working in the Earth, you experience a meditative reception within your 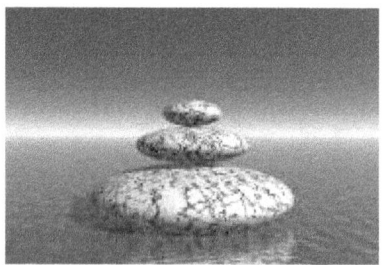 body that's different from what happens when you're indoors.

Some scientists believe the reason for the meditative association with nature has to do with the work involved in gardening. Preparing the soil for plants or flowers offers a repetitive task that allows the mind to free itself from the busy chaos and chatter of daily life.

It gives you a sense of happiness and a feeling of letting go while you work the soil. Studies also show that the work in your garden produces feel good hormones because it's a form of exercise from the smallest to the largest accomplishment.

Not only does handling the soil help you achieve a meditative state, but so does handling the plant. One of the reasons for this is due to all the greenery that you're surrounded with.

The color green symbolizes growth as well as healing, which automatically relaxes the mind. It boosts your mental well-being and makes you feel joy despite whatever stress you have going on in your life.

Being in nature can help you clear your mind because the greenery boosts your immune health, which in turn keeps sickness at bay. So you feel good physically and when you feel good physically, you feel better mentally and emotionally.

Having the hobby of gardening is known to relieve things like headaches, upset stomach, mood swings and more because of its ability to relieve stress. When you find relief from stress, it's easier to maintain a meditative state of mind.

Any time that you feel stressed or on edge about something, go outside and start working in the gardening. You'll feel better quickly and the things that are bothering you won't weigh so heavily on you.

Finding the Solace in Gardening

Even if you're single and live by yourself, it can be hard to focus on relaxation. That's because life is almost like one giant to-do list. You can't take days on end off from your life because there's always something that has to be handled.

You'll always have responsibilities - taking care of yourself, your pets, working your job, doing home repairs, taking care of your vehicle or handling transportation issues, getting groceries, cleaning, visiting the doctor or dentist.

The list is never-ending. With the workload, both physical and mental, that people have to deal with, it's why doctors recommend finding stress relief to prevent or cure health issues that stem from stress.

You have to find a way to clear your mind and free it from stress if you want to have a long, healthy life. You have to have mental downtime in order to recuperate. Most people don't get that.

It's one of the reasons that stress is so prevalent in today's society. Whether you're alone or not in gardening isn't as important as you finding peace in what you're doing. It's the peace and the focus that helps you achieve a state of mental relaxation.

When you get in touch with nature, you'll find that you distance yourself from the mental buzz that often comes with living a busy life. You're always "plugged in," always having to take care of stuff and not having a time out to recharge leads to compounding stress and mental clutter.

You need time by yourself even if you only have that time mentally. You can use gardening to achieve relaxation. You can't reach the point of relaxation if you don't free yourself from the mental noise and stress.

That's what gardening will give you. It will allow you to stop and get off the never-ending busy hamster wheel of demands. These demands clamor for your time and for your complete attention.

When you garden, you get to stop the hamster wheel and live in the moment for as long as you're in nature. Studies relating to relaxation and mental health have shown that out of all the hobbies you can engage in, gardening ranks number one as the most effective for achieving mental relaxation.

In fact, gardening can give you relief from stress and help you find peace faster than exercising does. The repetitive, relaxing state of gardening works to drop your levels of stress hormones, too.

So you feel better and have more energy to boot. Plus, you'll be able to enjoy the fruits of your labor at harvest time with all the lovely flowers or delicious foods you'll have grown yourself.

Gardening Helps You Focus

Many articles talk about the bonus of reaching the harvest point of gardening, but for those who are looking for mental relaxation gardening is a process. Rather than ending up with the harvest as your benefit, you reap a reduction in stress and a greater ability to focus.

One of the big issues with achieving mental relaxation is that you have to be able to clear your mind in order to focus. If you can't focus, it's much harder to achieve a point of complete mind relaxation.

Too many things are trying to butt in for you to quiet them all unless you know how to focus. If you've tried mental relaxation exercises in the past, then you know it can be difficult to completely clear your mind.

There's simply too much going on and each person will have a different amount of mind interruptions and different types of these interruptions. It's hard because we've conditioned ourselves to go 24/7 and it can become a habit to not be able to turn off the mind and go to sleep.

While that kind of burning the midnight oil drive might allow you to get a lot of things accomplished in your life, eventually, you'll burn out physically and mentally. No one can keep up a frantic pace without a point of stopping to decompress.

Your body simply won't let you push it beyond a certain point. That's why you need to do something that can help you with relaxation, something that can help you learn how to focus - such as gardening.

The beauty found in a garden and the way that the scents of nature appeal to the senses also help you to be able to clear your mind, which aids in helping you focus. When you focus, you achieve awareness and it allows you to pay attention to your inner thoughts and feelings.

This is important because many problems in life are rooted in how we think and feel. These can become conditioned patterns that cause us to react to stress in ways that are detrimental to our life goals and our personal happiness.

When you practice concentrated focus and follow peaceful meditation through gardening, it lets you stop allowing issues in your life to be at the forefront. Gardening offers you a break from stress by giving your creative side a way to develop with nature.

When you learn how to use gardening to help you focus so that you relax mentally, it will aid you in all the other areas of your life. People that know how to relax for increased focus are known to meet their goals easier than other people.

It allows you to be able to concentrate better on the things you want to accomplish in life. Plus, it gives you the ability to be happier while you're doing whatever it is you're pursuing.

Benefits You Gain by Using Gardening for Mental Relaxation

When you achieve mental relaxation, there's plenty of reward found in that. You feel better emotionally. When you don't have a way to find mental relaxation, you feel on edge all the time.

You can have higher levels of irritability. You might find it's easier to walk away in frustration rather than take care of stuff or deal with people. Gaining mental relaxation through gardening can help you because you'll be able to reach a more thoughtful way of dealing with issues.

When you do that, you'll notice that your level of anxiety is lower. The things that were once big enough to cause you to get upset either won't seem like a big deal or you'll have an easier time dealing with them.

That's because when you're not stressed mentally, you can handle things in a calmer manner. You won't immediately react to the emotion of the situation or to the person, but rather you'll be able to concentrate on the core problem and resolve it.

You'll learn how to be fully present in your life as a benefit of gardening for mental relaxation. With the meditation mindset you can find through gardening, you'll learn to stop and really experience life at that moment rather than letting it happen all around you.

You won't be a bystander anymore - you'll be a participant. You'll feel the moistness of the soil through your fingers. You'll hear the sound of the water as it gives the plants the hydration they need.

Experiencing these things in nature help you to connect with nature, move you to relax and let go of tension. Gardening benefits you gain also include finding harmony between your body and your mind.

It gives you a way to reflect inwardly and creates an opening for you to experience gratitude. As you observe the cycle of growth and life in gardening, it helps you be able to regain a state of being mindful of what's going on around you and within you.

You'll learn how to pour yourself into the moment that you're living. It's this process that lets you reach a state of natural meditation and your mind and body gain the same benefits from it as if you were actively engaging in practiced meditation habits. You'll feel your body's energy and zest for life restored through gardening.

The Natural Way to Reach Mental Relaxation

There are all kinds of practices that people will attempt in order to find relief from stress. Some people will turn to food. Others turn to activities that let them blank out such as mindlessly watching television.

Some people don't want to deal with things that bother them so they live in a state of having that nagging stress at the back of their minds, unable to relax completely. People want to achieve mental relaxation and so they'll seek avenues to help that often aren't good for their bodies.

Some people will attempt to find relief through the use of medications that have unpleasant side effects. Others will try to find relief by seeking out mind numbing alternatives, anything to disconnect from the stress they're living under.

The problem is that when you seek to find mental relaxation through unnatural methods, it's only a temporary fix. As soon as the effects of whatever you're using wear off, you'll feel the same or even worse than you did in the beginning.

It's always better to choose a more natural method in order to achieve mental relaxation. Gardening can give you this and you won't need to resort to any artificial means.

It doesn't matter if you spend a few minutes a day gardening or hours each day, you'll still find the peace you're seeking. That's because nature itself works to help you get to that meditative point.

When you work in a garden, you'll be out in the sun. Even if you carefully cover your head with a hat and put on sunscreen, you'll still gain the benefits of boosting your serotonin level.

When the serotonin level is increased, you'll experience an upswing in your emotions. You'll feel happier and less anxious. Being outside and experiencing the stillness of the day or the gentle breeze is beneficial toward achieving mental relaxation because it boosts your energy as well as helps to get rid of insomnia.

RON KNESS

You also get a boost in your vitamin D level. This vitamin, which is also called the sunshine vitamin, is necessary for you to feel good emotionally. When you're outside working in the garden, you gain the ability to be able to center yourself.

This allows you to put everything else in perspective and regain control over the stress that seems like it'll never end.

Gardening to Boost Your Immune System During Stress

Having a garden can be a work of art. You can plant beautiful flowers that can blossom with color all year round. Or you can have lush, delicious foods that you grow yourself. Your garden will be a haven for you, but more than that, it can give your immune system a boost.

You'd be surprised at all of the benefits your immune system can gain from spending time in a garden. It's a great form of exercise, which helps gives your body a surge of energy and hormone release.

Avoid the Hygiene Hypothesis Through Gardening

There are all sorts of warnings out on staying healthy. These warnings contain a laundry list of what you should avoid so that you don't get sick, you protect your immune system and you don't become burdened with stress.

The Hygiene Hypothesis is based in the belief that you can live a life so free of bacteria and illnesses that it actually worsens your immune system. You end up catching whatever it is that's going around because your immune system isn't strong enough.

When you add stress to the picture, your immune system undergoes even more depletion and it gets harder and harder to bounce back each time you get sick - each time you get stressed out.

The reason that all of this is coming to a head in today's society is that we're living in a world that's worked hard to eradicate anything that can make us sick. Because of that, our immune systems don't have a chance to flex their muscles, so to speak.

Any muscle, any part of your body that's not activated on a regular basis, will automatically become weaker. When your immune system isn't put to the test, when it isn't pushed into activation mode, it doesn't work as well.

It becomes puny. The eroding of the immune system is caused by the cleanliness in which we live our lives. There is hand soap containing anti-bacterial agents. Shampoos that fight bacteria can be purchased.

Antibiotics are given before surgery "just in case" and they're prescribed by dentists and doctors to "ward off" anything that might make you sick. With the Hygiene Hypothesis, you'll see that studies show that the problem of not letting the immune system have a regular work out contributes to many illnesses and common ailments.

When you work hard to prevent bacteria and germs from touching your life, you're more at risk for things like allergies, asthma and skin conditions. Many studies suggest that the reason for the growing number of allergy diagnosis in kids is because the immune system doesn't get a chance to fight off things when it's over-protected.

When your system is over-protected, you can also end up having to fight the same illnesses repeatedly. When you add stress to the mix, your poor immune system just can't handle what's going on.

That's why you need to forget about avoiding every kind of bacteria - because not all of them are bad for you. In fact, some of the bacteria helps you and without it in your life, you simply won't be as strong and you won't be able to fight off illnesses or stress the way that it was intended for you to.

The Friendly Bacteria Living in Your Garden

If you played in the dirt as a kid, you might have heard your mom tell you to get out of the dirt. There was a negative connotation that not only did playing in the dirt mess up your clothes but that it could make you sick.

The reason that soil has gotten a bad rap over the years as being something to avoid is because it contains bacteria. There's a mindset that since bacteria is bad and lives in the dirt, then all bacteria living in the dirt should be left alone.

It's true that the dirt does contain bacteria, but it's not true that it's something to be avoided. There is friendly bacteria in the soil that actually boosts your immune system and can help protect you from illnesses as well as help you be able to deal with the symptoms of stress.

The friendly bacteria found in the soil is called mycobacterium vaccae. Unfortunately, not many people get to experience the helpful ability of this bacteria. It can strengthen the immune system in both children and adults.

This bacteria happens to be nonpathogenic, so it's not harmful to the body. Plus, the more often you come in contact with the friendly bacteria, the tougher your immune system will become.

Not only can the bacteria boost your immune system during times of stress, but it can also be used to help keep depression at bay.

It does this because the bacteria works to help boost the amount of serotonin that your body produces.

Serotonin works as a neurotransmitter and is connected to helping the function of cells - including the cells that help you with how you feel. So, this chemical acting as a neurotransmitter is boosted by the bacteria that you'll find in dirt.

When you get this boost, you feel better as far as your moods go. It's a healthier, more natural way to boost your immune system during stress than it is to take stress relieving medications.

So when you decide that you're going to take up the hobby of gardening to help alleviate stress, there are all kinds of extra benefits just waiting to give your body a hand in feeling better.

Grow Superfoods to Boost Your Immune System

There are foods, then there are superfoods. Superfoods are foods that give you more healthy benefits than ordinary foods. Superfoods are loaded with vitamins and minerals that are known to boost the immune system.

Not only that, but they're foods that can help to protect your body from illnesses and diseases when you're stressed. You might know that making sure you have fruits in your everyday eating plan is a good idea.

However, some fruits are more powerful than others are because they're superfoods. Blueberries happen to be one of the superfoods.

This tasty little berry actually works to reduce stress.

Not only is it a healthy addition to your diet but it's jam packed with antioxidants, which work to keep you healthy and fight off illnesses. But that's not all that blueberries can do.

These delightful fruits are known to help lower stress and alleviate the symptoms most often associated with stress. Plus, the berries can help you with mood stability. They're known to calm irritation, smooth out moods that make you feel anxious and can even battle the side effects that are associated with depression.

These berries are low maintenance foods to grow so they don't take a lot of time or effort to bring them to harvest. You can plant several blueberry bushes anywhere in your yard.

Oranges are another superfood that you'll want to add to your garden. Many people are surprised to discover that oranges can be grown right in their own backyard. You may have thought that oranges were grown mostly in places with a lot of sunshine like Florida or California.

But you can grow oranges anywhere. You just have to make sure you watch them closely for pests and that you keep them moist - especially during the summer months when it's easier for the trees to dry out.

Some people start with dwarf orange trees. These fruits are packed full of antioxidants as well as vitamins and minerals that boost your immune system. They contain vitamin C which is a well-known stress buster that can help your body stay healthy both physically and emotionally.

One of the easiest superfoods that you can grow in your garden is an avocado. These superfoods are loaded with vitamins and minerals as well as being packed with potassium.

The ingredients in an avocado help your body with stress because they stabilize the hormones that regulate the stress. When you eat them, they get to work to lower the amount of stress hormones you have in your body so you feel the effects.

Plus, they're also known to bring blood pressure levels down, which can also help make you feel less stressed. It's easy to grow an avocado right from the seed. You have to put the seed in just a little bit of water until it sprouts roots.

Once you have roots and a stem from the seed, you can plant the seed in your garden. You'll need a lot of sunshine, but other than minimal moisture, the food grows fairly well on its own.

Another superfood that you can grow in your garden to help boost your immune system is spinach. Like other superfoods, it's loaded with vitamins and minerals. But it also contains magnesium.

This mineral is vital in helping to lower the amount of stress hormones that your body produces when you're feeling stressed. On top of that, it works to ease the anxiety that you feel when you get stressed.

It doesn't take a lot of this superfood to give you that healthy benefit either. A healthy diet of this stress buster will have you consuming about a cup full with your eating plan. Spinach is easy to use in dishes and it's easy to grow in the garden because it's hardy and grows fast.

You can choose either smooth or savoyed leaf varieties for your garden to gain the stress beating benefits the food offers. Tomatoes are another superfood that you can grow right in your own garden and this food is a great stress buster.

They're full of vitamins and minerals like vitamin C, A and E as well as loaded with vitamins from the B family. They contain antioxidants, particularly lycopene, which helps your body reduce your risk of developing certain cancers.

Not only can lycopene help you live longer, it also lowers stress. You'll also want to make sure that your garden contains asparagus which is a popular superfood. This vegetable is loaded with vitamins and minerals but more importantly, it contains a lot of folic acid.

Folic acid is known as a mood stabilizer as well as a mood booster because they aid the body in the production of serotonin that can help to relieve the symptoms of stress. When you plant asparagus crowns, it's always better to plant them in a raised bed and plant them about a foot or two apart for best results.

Asparagus is a hardy vegetable that doesn't take a lot of monitoring to grow well. Finally, you'll also want to make sure that you grow kale in your garden. This superfood is one of the top immune system boosters when it comes to helping the body handle stress.

It's loaded with antioxidants including vitamin C. The food is widely known for its ability to fight off the free radicals that cause damage to the body as well as open you up to diseases.

You can easily grow the plant regardless of when you plant it. You need to make sure it has sunshine in the cooler temperatures and shade in the summer temperatures along with moist but not saturated soil.

You Get Vitamin D with Gardening

Most people think that they get plenty of vitamin D when they drink milk or eat dairy products that contain the vitamin. But vitamin D deficiencies are on the rise and it's tied in to how your body deals with stress.

Whenever you're under stress, your body starts working to produce cortisol. The more stressed that you are, the more cortisol that you produce. This cycle then affects your vitamin D or rather the way that your body can use the amount of the vitamin that you get.

When there's more cortisol production in the body, it prohibits the vitamin from being absorbed. So regardless of how much vitamin D you get in milk or dairy products, your body isn't getting any of the healthy benefits from it.

With a lack of the right amount of vitamin D, you'll start to feel the effects. A lack of vitamin D has been linked to asthma. It also causes a higher rate of depression because the body isn't producing the right amount of serotonin.

When you don't have the right amount of serotonin, you're more at risk for depression and other emotional upsets. Without a healthy serotonin production, you'll feel more stressed and the symptoms may be worse.

Fortunately, there's a way to stop the body from producing high amounts of cortisol that cause you to stay stressed. You have to get vitamin D and it needs to be absorbed in greater amounts and easier.

The best way to do that is to get outside and start gardening. When you spend time gardening, it relaxes you, allowing the cortisol level to drop.

As the cortisol level drops, your body is able to absorb the amount of vitamin D that you get from being out in the sunshine.

With the absorption of sunshine, your immune system gets a boost even if you've been dealing with chronic stress. The benefits of gardening on your immune system shouldn't be overlooked. Not only is gardening easy and low cost, but it can provide you with healthy foods, a healthier body and a mind that's at peace more often than not.

Stress Relieving Gardening Techniques

John Burroughs, a writer and naturalist from America, once said, "I go to nature to be soothed and healed, and to have my senses put in tune once more."

Since ancient times, gardening has been known as a natural stress reliever. Today, healthcare providers consistently recommend gardening activities to patients struggling with issues that are negatively affecting all aspects of their lives.

The activity itself, plus enjoying the peace, beauty and bounty of gardening can lower stress levels and promote health and wellness in your life. Even if you don't have a huge garden space in your backyard, gardening activities are readily available for you.

New and innovative techniques have made it possible for anyone who lives anywhere to enjoy the beauty, peace and wellness that gardening can provide. You're about to discover the most popular techniques in today's gardening world: hydroponic, container, tower, raised bed and bottle gardening.

By the time you reach the end of the report, you'll be anxious to start on one or all of these stress-relieving – and fun – techniques.

Hydroponic Gardening – A Year-Round, Relaxing Hobby

If you're anxious to get into gardening, but lack an outdoor space to grow anything significant, hydroponic gardening may be an option you want to pursue. If you've ever stuck a cutting from a plant in a glass of water to root, you've practiced the art of hydroponic gardening.

It's a hobby that can provide you with many hours of relaxing, stress-free activities – plus, provide you with beautiful, healthy food for the table. It's a soilless method that uses enriched water to produce heathy plants.

The name, "hydroponic," means "working water" and you can achieve many benefits which can't be accomplished by normal gardening with soil. You'll get faster growth, more yields to the plantings and use less water to hydrate the plants than soil.

Although you won't have to get your hands dirty, you'll have the mind-soothing benefits of planning your garden, setting up the hydroponic growing area, tending and growing the plants.

Hydroponic kits are available at most garden outlets or home improvement stores (or online). 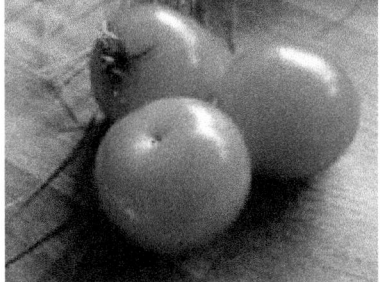 There are also instructions available so you can make your own. Choose the system according to the amount of space you can devote.

If the room you choose is small, keep the door or window open for the correct amount of air as plants breathe in all of the CO_2 (carbon dioxide) in the room.

A fan works perfectly, but make sure it blows away from the plants.

Light may be hard to come by for hours at a time in an indoor area, so you'll need supplemental lighting. Indoor grow lights are available in all sizes and shapes and easy to come by.

Humidity is very important for your hydroponic garden. If you don't have the proper amount, it can ruin your gardening efforts. You'll want to keep the air-conditioning in the area of the garden at between 72 and 76 degrees or purchase a small A/C window unit for the room.

Now that you're equipped and ready to grow, it's time to create a relaxing space for yourself – so you can enjoy your efforts. Create a space for yourself by choosing a comfy chair to observe and even talk to your plants as you would a counselor.

Scientific studies have proven that plants that are spoken to thrive more than plants left in a silent environment. They're not quite sure why yet, but it might help alleviate your stress knowing that using them as a sounding board is helping them grow!

Train them on trellises and use a magnifying glass to search for and destroy bugs, which may be detrimental to the health and growth of the plants. Enjoy a good book while resting in your growing room or relax with some soft music. The plants will love it and you'll find amazing stress relief.

Container Gardening – Little Effort with Big Results

Connecting with the earth is an important part of staying calm, cool and stress-free. If you live in a bubble of life containing stressful thoughts and activities, you'll miss the natural rhythms that can ultimately keep your stress levels down.

Gardening is one way to connect with the earth. You may not have acreage for a farm or even a plot for a high-yield vegetable garden, but you may have a patio or sunny spot in your home for container gardening.

Digging, pruning and realizing the bounty of what you've done – whether for beauty or food – can be a great outlet for tension and frustration that's built up over time in your body and mind.

By tending your container garden and watching it grow, you'll be struck by what is important in your life – love, water, space and warmth. It's easy to forget those things as you muddle through life's busy schedules.

Bringing them back to the forefront of your life helps you focus on what's real and important. Container gardening is a good way for you to begin your gardening journey small and then work up to a plot in the yard or more spacious containers for your plants.

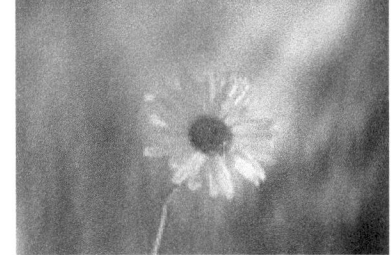

Plant what makes you happy – flowers or fragrant herbs are good beginnings to any garden space.

Besides the physical activity that gardening provides, you'll gain flexibility and your lungs and heart will become stronger.

Weight control is an added benefit. You're more likely to eat what you grow and the fresh taste will make you want to eat healthier. Studies indicate that a regular type of physical activity can lessen your chances of premature death and keep you from developing heart disease, diabetes, cancer, depression and high blood pressure.

Gardening provides a path for you to get physical activity in your life in a meaningful and joyful way. If you've never gardened before, container gardening is a good place to begin.

Start small, with a few pots and some easy plants to grow. Flowers can make you feel happy and add beauty to your space. Herbs and vegetables bring heavenly scents into your life and add color and creativeness to meals.

Don't worry about being a perfectionist. Just begin and then sit back and enjoy what you've created. A patio space, balcony or porch makes wonderful areas for a container garden.

Then, choose your containers from pots you already have or purchase some special, decorative pots for your garden. You can find tons of information online and in "container gardening" books.

Whether you start from seeds or seedlings, you'll likely find more plants than you even have space for as a beginning to your gardening journey. You may want to create a space just for you among your overflowing containers.

A small water feature can add much to the ambiance of calmness. The sound is soothing. Take breaks throughout the day or evening and enjoy the space you've brought to life.

Tower Gardening for Small Spaces

If you want to try gardening as a way to relieve stress and enjoy the beauty and bounty that a garden brings to your life, but feel you don't have the space – consider tower gardening.

Tower gardening has become the trend in gardening. As our lives become more and more confined to smaller spaces, gardening may seem to be out of reach, but with tower gardening, you can enjoy all the aspects of gardening – without a ton of space.

This type of gardening is one answer to the "lack of space" problem. Your plants are set to grow in a vertical, rather than horizontal, space and it works beautifully. With tower gardening, you still get the benefits of relaxation and freedom from stress – plus the beauty and harvest that a garden provides.

Tower gardening is also for those of us who lack the ubiquitous "green thumb" – or the time necessary to tend to a sizeable garden plot. A simple way to explain tower gardening is that it's an aeroponic/hydroponic, vertical method of growing plants.

All you need is a sunny place on a rooftop, balcony or patio. The "tower of plants" rise to about five feet tall and about 2 ½ feet wide – and you can grow as many as twenty plants at once.

Herbs, flowers, melons, tomatoes, peas and other veggies can be grown fresh and without chemicals for your dining enjoyment. You don't have to lug bags of soil because a tower garden is grown without it.

It's a completely water-based system. Nutrients in the water and air are all you need to feed and nourish the plants. If you have trouble kneeling and bending, you'll be happy to know that tower gardening doesn't require it.

Information about tower gardening can be found online or in books. Your local gardening store can also be a wealth of information you can call on. Tower gardening is a great way to get all the benefits gardening can bring into your life without the space or the usual hassles of creating a soil-based garden.

When you finish planting and creating your tower garden, sit back, relax and watch it grow. It's a fascinating way to garden.

Raised Bed Gardening Can Lower Health Risks

Gardening is proven to be one of the best stress relievers and health boosters you can engage in. It provides exercise which releases vital serotonin from the brain to help boost your mood – and can reduce the risk of health problems such as obesity, adult diabetes and high blood pressure.

You may have steered away from gardening as an exercise and stress reliever because of not being able to meet the physical rigors of bending, lifting and other physical requirements.

Or, you may not think you have enough space for a garden. Raised bed gardening is the solution – both for space and any physical disability you may have. They're simple garden boxes, raised from ground level to provide easy access to tending and also act as protection from pests such as snails and slugs.

This type of gardening also provides excellent drainage for your plants, preventing root rot or garden soil from being washed away during storms and heavy rain. The containers are bottomless and open to the soil so the plants' roots can push further into the ground for nutrients.

You can sit on the side of the bed while planting, weeding and harvesting and enjoy the health and other benefits of gardening without the back strain from bending. You can build your own or purchase the right size for you and your plants from any gardening facility – or online.

They come in a number of sizes and types – the cedar-made raised beds being the highest quality of wood and may prevent pests from feeding on your plants. The hardware that keeps it together is usually stainless steel and some even 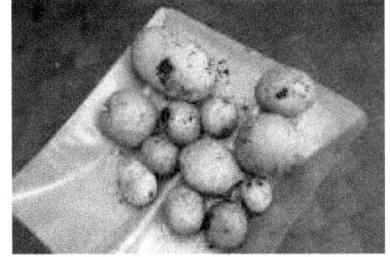 have decorative posts to prevent a garden hose from sliding across your delicate plants.

You can create a garden spot with raised garden beds which

add ambiance and beauty to any outdoor space. Grow a variety of plants for beauty and food and you'll reap the benefits in health and in a serene and beautiful place to relax.

Bottle Gardening – More Than Decoration

Bottle gardening has been a growing trend since the early 1960s (the first notification) and was used mainly for decorative purposes. Usually planted in a glass or plastic bottle, the enclosed, ecological environment is perfect to grow plants – as long as it gets the proper amount of light exposure.

A bottle garden resembles a terrarium, but bottles usually have slim necks and narrow openings. The plants have very little exposure to the environment outside the bottle and are perfect for apartments, patios and balconies.

Schools sometimes use bottle gardens to demonstrate how eco-systems work and are super-easy to maintain. Even though it's a small area in which to garden, bottle gardens can provide the same relaxation and stress relief therapy as a full garden in a large space.

Create as many bottle gardens as you like and enjoy the observation of this near-maintenance-free environment that produces plants for food and beauty. Any bottle will do – plastic or glass.

Online ideas for bottle gardening beginners exist in abundance and can be a great source of fun for the entire family.

If you're a gardener who gets bored during the winter months, this type of gardening can keep you busy.

It's easy. All you need to do is select your bottle (make sure it's large enough for the plant you choose), clean it thoroughly and dry it. Also, make sure it has a large enough opening to maintain the contents.

With the bottle right side up, add stones and sand to provide drainage for the plants. Add some activated charcoal on top of the mixture to prevent fungus and smell within the bottle.

Then, add the soil. Consider a thin layer of sphagnum moss on top to further help the drainage. Small, indoor plant seeds are best for bottle gardens (especially those which need a great amount of humidity).

Using a stick or tweezers, carefully plant the seeds in the soil. Now, sit back and watch the miracle of life occur. Bottle gardening is an ideal way to break into gardening as a hobby if you've never done it before.

It's a fun an easy way to connect with nature, but begin in a way that doesn't take too much time and effort. Remember that any type of gardening is good for the body and soul.

Your psychological and emotional well-being can be greatly enhanced by choosing a gardening activity that you enjoy and one which will nurture you in every way. You'll enjoy a serene environment that helps connect you with nature and ease away from the hurried and hectic of your world today.

Other Senior Health and Fitness Books by THis Author

If you would like to read more about Senior Health and Fitness, here is a list of the <u>titles, CreateSpace links and descriptions:</u>

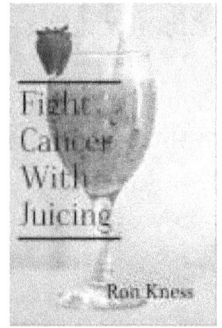

<u>Fight Cancer With Juicing</u>

https://www.createspace.com/6155567

Juicing is a healthy practice that has allowed millions of people to boost their nutrition. Juicing fruits and vegetables provides you important antioxidants, which scavenge for oxygen free radicals that can damage cellular structures, including DNA. When DNA is damaged, it can result in mutations that lead to cancer.

Well-balanced nutrition from a variety of healthy whole foods helps support and maintain on-going good health, and experts agree that nutrition plays a key role in preventing chronic and terminal illness.

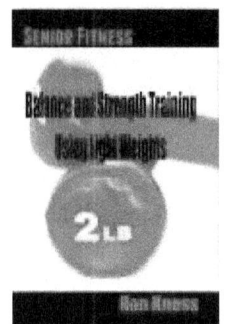

<u>Senior Fitness – Balance and Strength Training Using Light Weights</u>

https://www.createspace.com/6107842

As you age you notice that you are not as strong as before. Most of us simply chalk that up to the "natural" aging process. However, to fight the physical dangers of aging, strength is very important.

We are not talking about bodybuilding and packing on bulky muscles. What we mean is simply making your body stronger so that you don't become a statistic.

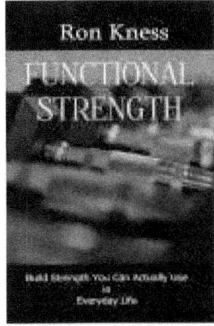

Functional Strength – Build Strength You Can Actually Use
https://www.createspace.com/6114822

Health and fitness fads come and go all the time but unfortunately not all of them are worth your time and effort. Some of them don't work, some of them are over-hyped and some of them are just plain dangerous.

But 'functional strength' is different. While functional strength is very much in vogue right now, it's not a 'fad' by any means. In fact, functional strength is the opposite of a fad and it's a step in the right direction for all of fitness.

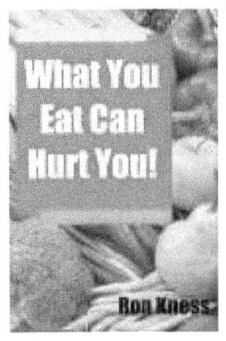

What You Eat Can Hurt You

https://www.createspace.com/4963196

Do you know that certain foods increase your risk for inflammation, disease and illness? It's true! And certain foods can help cure and heal you if you do get sick. Knowing which foods to eat and which ones to avoid empowers you to manage your own health.

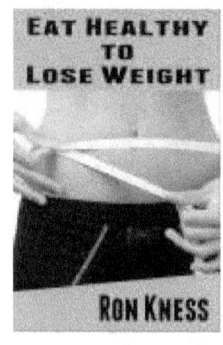

Eat Healthy to Lose Weight

https://www.createspace.com/4962939

As you read through our book, we show you which foods you should and should not be eating to reach your weight loss goal, along with discussing how to maintain your weight loss and stay within a few pounds of your goal weight. Banish the weight you keep gaining back each time by learning how to live a healthy lifestyle.

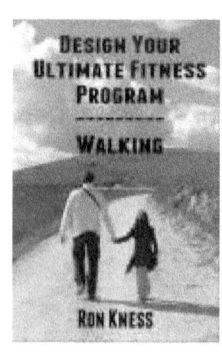

Design Your Ultimate Fitness Program - Walking

https://www.createspace.com/5252272

In my book Design Your Ultimate Fitness Program – Walking, we discuss the considerations that need to be made when designing a custom walking program, along with:

• Equipment needed
• Wearable technology you can use to track your walking
• And how to make walking more challenging

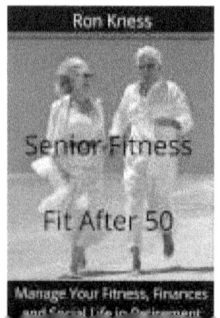

Senior Fitness – Fit After 50: Learn How to Manage Your Fitness, Finances and Social Life in Retirement

https://www.createspace.com/5474751

Inside you will discover answers to your most pressing questions:
• What do I need to know about downsizing my home?
• What are the best tips for staying healthy as you approach your 50's?
• When should I start planning for retirement?
• I am worried about being lonely once I retire, do others feel the same?
• Is it worthwhile to carry two homes during retirement?
And more…

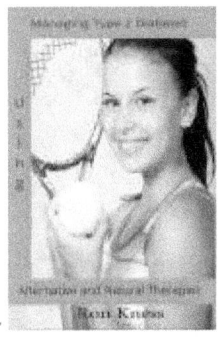

Managing Type 2 Diabetes Using Alternative And Natural Therapies

https://www.createspace.com/5401244

While Type 2 diabetes can be managed medically, there are many alternative natural and holistic methods of therapy and treatment that can further enhance quality of life and minimize the effects of this disease. In this book, I discuss 12 different types, including yoga, reflexology and acupuncture to name just three.

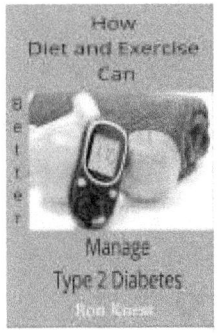

How Diet and Exercise Can Better Manage Type 2 Diabetes

https://www.createspace.com/5404845

Of the different types of diabetes, only Type 2 can be reversed. In my book How Diet and Exercise Can Better Manage Type 2 Diabetes,

we reveal the three things you can do to best manage your disease, including:
• Diet
• Exercise
• Weight management

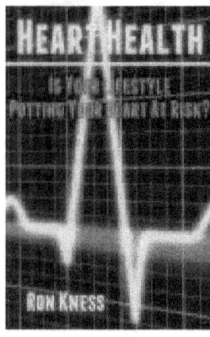

Heart Health: Is Your Lifestyle Putting Your Heart at Risk?

https://www.createspace.com/5464020

In my ebook Is Your Lifestyle Putting Your Heart At Risk? we discuss the six greatest risks to your heart and the lifestyle changes you can make to mitigate them.

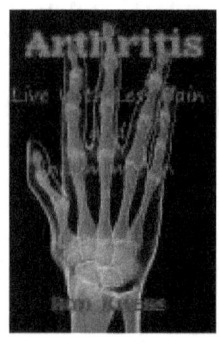

Arthritis – Live Wth Less Pain and Inflammation: Tips and Techniques You Can Use to Lessen the Pain and Inflammation

https://www.createspace.com/5457441

Discover Simple Tips & Information That Will Help Reduce The Painful Symptoms Of Arthritis!

You learn things like:
• Simple and effective information that will help you manage the pain and inflammation that comes along with arthritis, so that you can live an active, full life without debilitating pain.
• The different types of arthritis, their symptoms and how to alleviate their painful side effects.

• The pros and cons of over-the-counter arthritis medications, plus simple tips that will help you know how to choose the right supplements.

• Free, yet effective ways to get relief from arthritis pain and inflammation, so you don't have to suffer anymore.

the effects arthritis can have significant impact on your physical and mental well-being, but this books shows you how to overcome its painful symptoms and live life relatively pain free.

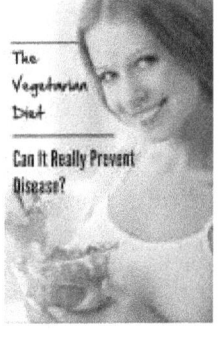

The Vegetarian Diet – Can It Really Prevent Disease?

https://www.createspace.com/5519874

Is a vegetarian diet right for you? Multiple studies have shown over and over that a vegetarian diet goes along way in preventing certain chronic diseases, such as:

• Heart Disease
• Cancer
• Diverticulitis
• Type 2 Diabetes
• Hypertension
• Obesity
• Kidney Failure

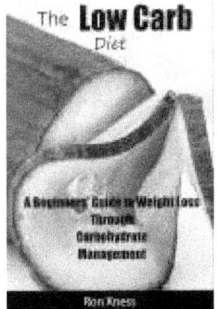

The Low Carb Diet: A Beginner's Guide to Weight Loss Through Carbohydrate Management

https://www.createspace.com/5416348

In my book "The Low-Carb Diet – A Beginners' Guide to Weight Loss Through Carbohydrate Management", I reveal a successful method of losing weight based in part on the amount and type of carbohydrates you consume.

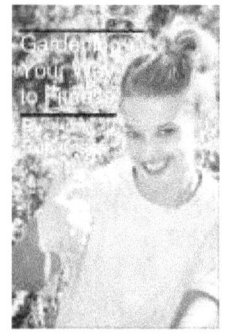

Gardening Your Way to Fitness: The Fun Way to Get Fit and Provide Beauty and Healthful Bounty for Your Family

https://www.createspace.com/5459564

The gym is a great place to stay fit during the colder seasons, but once the temperature turns warmer you want to spend more time outside. Plus, you'll have the benefit of fresh wholesome produce to enjoy by growing vegetables in your backyard garden.

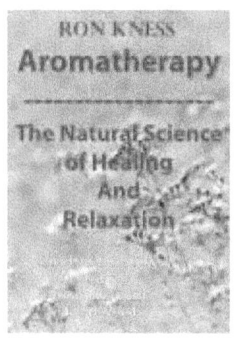

Aromatherapy - The Science of Healing and Relaxation: Learn How Essential Oils Elicit The Relaxation Response And Alter Mood

https://www.createspace.com/5714434

In my book Aromatherapy – The Science of Healing and Relaxation, we reveal the natural holistics methods you can use to heal the body from certain medical issues and to relive stress through relaxation. In particular we talk about:

• Aromatherapy - what it is and how it works

• Essential Oils – how the effects of certain aromas differs from others

• Recipes – how to make your own essential oil combinations

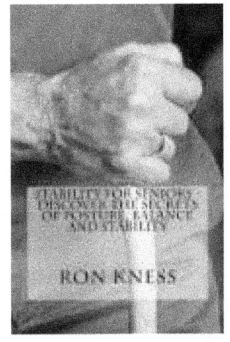

Stability for Seniors: Discover the Secrets of Posture, Balance and Stability

https://www.createspace.com/6096479

Many people sacrifice their health in pursuit of their career. They are so busy making a living that they neglect to make a life. The excuse that they do not have time to exercise is tossed about so frequently that they end up letting their health and fitness slide.

If you are not regularly active, you will have muscular atrophy over time. Your flexibility will decrease. Your core strength will diminish. As time progresses, you will be less limber and more rigid.

This is exactly how people age poorly. It's a process that has snowballed over time.

Only with regular exercise and a healthy diet can you have a body that is fit and has the ability to almost reverse aging.

If you have neglected your health for years and life seems to be a chore now because you can't get around without assistance, do not feel dejected.

You can remedy the situation. You can restore the strength, balance and stamina that you have lost. It is never too late to become what you might have been.

This guide will show you exactly what you need to do to restore your balance, strengthen your core and give you the ability to live life to its fullest. Read how …

About the Author

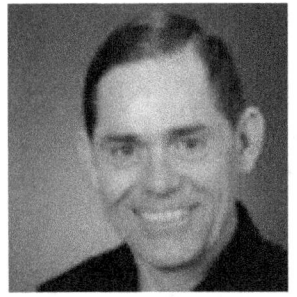

I grew up in Central Minnesota, where my parents own and operated a fishing resort. Once out of high school I tried a couple of semesters of college, only to quit halfway through the Spring term; I decided at that time that college wasn't for me.

Then I decided to follow my father's previous occupation as an auto mechanic. I graduated from a two-year of vocational training course and worked as a mechanic. While in vocational training, I decided to join the National Guard where I eventually ended up working full-time for 32 years.

So how does all of this relate to writing? In one of my leadership schools, the instructor, who was an English teacher at a juvenile detention center, presented writing to me in a whole new way - a way that started to develop my interest in working with words.

Fast forward about 40 years and I now have over 50 books listed on Amazon for Kindle and Createspace.

Today my wife and I live in Gold Canyon, AZ, where you'll find me happily sitting in my office typing away on my laptop as I work on my next book or ghostwriting project . . . that is if we are not traveling on a cruise ship - our new-found mode of travel.

If you like my book, please leave a review of it.

www.ingramcontent.com/pod-product-compliance
Lightning Source LLC
Chambersburg PA
CBHW071239280526
45787CB00002B/993